Why This Book?

This book aims to demystify art therapy and provide readers with a comprehensive understanding of its principles, methods, and benefits. Whether you are a mental health professional looking to incorporate art therapy into your practice, a student aspiring to become an art therapist, or an individual seeking new ways to enhance your personal well-being, this book will serve as a valuable resource. We will explore the theoretical foundations of art therapy, present practical techniques and activities, and share real-life case studies to illustrate the transformative power of art.

A Journey of Self-Discovery and Healing

Embarking on the journey of art therapy is both an exploration and a discovery. It invites you to tap into your creative potential and uncover the depths of your inner world. Through this process, you can gain clarity, find meaning, and experience healing in ways that are both profound and enduring. As you read through the chapters of this book, I encourage you to keep an open mind and heart, allowing the creative process to guide you towards greater self-awareness and emotional resilience.

Welcome to the world of art therapy. May this book inspire you, inform you, and, most importantly, empower you to harness the healing power of art.

This introduction sets the stage for your book, providing readers with an overview of what art therapy is, its historical context, and the benefits it offers. It also outlines the purpose of the book and invites readers to engage with the material in a meaningful way.

Chapter 2: Understanding the Art Therapy

Art therapy is a unique blend of psychology and the creative process, designed to enhance the mental, emotional, and physical well-being of individuals. It uses the creation of art to help people explore their emotions, develop self-awareness, cope with stress, boost self-esteem, and work through traumatic experiences. This chapter will delve into the core principles and theoretical foundations of art therapy, providing a deeper understanding of how and why it works.

Definition and Scope

Art therapy is defined by the American Art Therapy Association as a mental health profession that uses the creative process of art-making to improve and enhance the physical, mental, and emotional well-being of individuals. It is based on the belief that the creative process involved in artistic self-expression helps people resolve conflicts and problems, develop interpersonal skills, manage behavior, reduce stress, increase self-esteem and self-awareness, and achieve insight.

Theoretical Foundations

Art therapy draws from various psychological theories and approaches, integrating them into its practice. Here are some of the primary theories that inform art therapy:

Psychoanalytic and Psychodynamic Theories: These approaches, pioneered by Sigmund Freud and Carl Jung, emphasize the importance of the unconscious mind and early childhood experiences. In art therapy, creating art can be a way to access and express unconscious thoughts and feelings. Jung's concept of archetypes and the collective unconscious can be explored through symbolic imagery in art.

Humanistic Theories: Influenced by Carl Rogers and Abraham Maslow, humanistic approaches focus on the individual's capacity for self-actualization and personal growth. Art therapy in this context is client-centered, emphasizing empathy, unconditional positive regard, and the therapist's role in providing a supportive environment for creative expression.

Welcome to "The Art of Healing: Exploring Art Therapy for Personal Growth and Emotional Well-Being."

In the midst of life's challenges and complexities, we all seek avenues for understanding, healing, and personal growth. Art therapy offers a unique and profound way to explore these needs through the power of creative expression. This book is a journey into the transformative world of art therapy, where colors, shapes, and textures become tools for self-discovery, emotional release, and healing.

Whether you are a seasoned artist or someone who has never picked up a paintbrush, this book invites you to delve into the therapeutic potential of art. Here, you will find not only the theoretical foundations of art therapy but also practical exercises, inspiring case studies, and thoughtful reflections on the role of creativity in our lives.

Art therapy transcends the boundaries of traditional verbal therapy. It taps into the nonverbal language of the heart and mind, allowing for the expression of thoughts and feelings that words often cannot capture. Through the process of creating art, we can uncover hidden parts of ourselves, gain insights into our experiences, and foster a deeper connection with our inner world.

In these pages, you will discover how art therapy can be applied to various aspects of personal growth and emotional well-being. From managing stress and anxiety to enhancing self-esteem and resolving trauma, the practices shared here are designed to guide you toward a more fulfilling and balanced life.

As you embark on this journey, remember that there is no right or wrong way to create art. The value lies in the process, not the product. Each stroke of the brush, each line drawn, and each color chosen is a step toward greater self-awareness and healing.

Thank you for choosing to explore the art of healing with me. I hope this book serves as a valuable resource and a source of inspiration on your path to personal growth and emotional well-being.

With creativity and compassion,

Shazia Naqib

Chapter 1: Introduction

In a world that often feels chaotic and overwhelming, finding avenues for self-expression and healing is more important than ever. Art therapy offers a unique and powerful way to explore and understand our inner lives, using the creative process to foster emotional resilience and personal growth. This book is a comprehensive guide to understanding and practicing art therapy, designed for both aspiring art therapists and individuals looking to incorporate art into their own healing journeys.

The Essence of Art Therapy

Art therapy is a therapeutic practice that combines the creative process of making art with the exploration of psychological and emotional experiences. Unlike traditional talk therapy, art therapy allows individuals to express feelings and thoughts that might be difficult to articulate with words alone. Through various art forms—such as drawing, painting, sculpture, and digital media—individuals can gain insights into their emotions, develop coping strategies, and work through trauma and stress.

The Origins and Evolution of Art Therapy

The roots of art therapy can be traced back to the mid-20th century, with pioneers like Margaret Naumburg and Edith Kramer who recognized the profound impact that art-making could have on mental health. Since then, art therapy has grown into a respected and widely practiced therapeutic discipline, grounded in both psychological theory and artistic practice. Today, art therapists work in a variety of settings, including hospitals, schools, rehabilitation centers, and private practices, helping people of all ages and backgrounds.

Who Can Benefit from Art Therapy?

Art therapy is incredibly versatile and can be beneficial for a wide range of populations. Children and adolescents often find it easier to express themselves through art than through words, making art therapy an effective tool for addressing developmental and emotional challenges. Adults, too, can use art therapy to navigate life's complexities, from coping with mental health issues to processing major life changes. Even the elderly can benefit from art therapy, using it to enhance cognitive function and emotional well-being in later life.

Cognitive-Behavioral Theories: Cognitive-behavioral approaches, such as those developed by Aaron Beck and Albert Ellis, focus on changing negative thought patterns and behaviors. Art therapy can be used to identify and alter cognitive distortions, using art-making as a means to practice new ways of thinking and behaving.

Developmental Theories: These theories, including those by Jean Piaget and Erik Erikson, focus on the stages of human development. Art therapy can help individuals at different developmental stages by providing age-appropriate ways to explore and express their experiences and emotions.

The Healing Power of Art

Art has the unique ability to transcend verbal communication, allowing individuals to express what may be difficult or impossible to put into words. The process of creating art can serve multiple therapeutic functions:

Expression: Art provides a safe outlet for expressing feelings and thoughts that may be repressed or unconscious. This can lead to a greater understanding of oneself and one's emotions.

Relaxation: Engaging in creative activities can induce a state of flow, reducing stress and promoting relaxation. The repetitive and rhythmic actions involved in many forms of art-making can be calming and meditative.

Problem-Solving: Art-making can help individuals externalize problems, allowing them to be examined from different perspectives. This can facilitate problem-solving and insight.

Empowerment: Creating art can boost self-esteem and self-efficacy, as individuals see tangible evidence of their abilities and creative potential.

Case Studies

To illustrate the impact of art therapy, consider the following case studies:

Case Study 1: Sarah's Journey Through Trauma

Sarah, a 35-year-old woman, sought art therapy to cope with past trauma. Through painting, she was able to express the pain and fear she had experienced, which she had found difficult to articulate in words. Over time, her artwork became a powerful tool for processing her trauma and reclaiming her sense of self. Through guided sessions, Sarah created a series of paintings that depicted her journey from darkness to light, symbolizing her healing process.

Case Study 2: Mark's Battle with Depression

Mark, a 22-year-old college student, struggled with severe depression. Traditional talk therapy had limited success, so his therapist suggested art therapy as a complementary approach. Mark began creating collages, which helped him externalize his feelings of despair and hopelessness. The process of selecting and arranging images allowed him to explore and challenge his negative thought patterns. Gradually, his collages began to reflect more hopeful and positive themes, mirroring his progress in therapy.

Art Therapy Modalities

Art therapy can incorporate a wide range of artistic modalities, each offering unique benefits:

Drawing and Painting: These are the most common forms of art used in therapy. They allow for immediate expression and can be adapted to various skill levels and therapeutic goals.

Sculpture and 3D Art: Working with clay, wood, or other materials can be particularly grounding and tactile, helping individuals connect with their physicality and creativity.

Collage and Mixed Media: Combining different materials and images can be a metaphor for bringing together disparate parts of oneself. Collage can be particularly useful for individuals who may feel fragmented or overwhelmed.

Digital Art: With the advent of technology, digital art has become an accessible and versatile tool in art therapy. It allows for endless experimentation and can be less intimidating for those who are uncomfortable with traditional art materials.

Photography: Photography can be a powerful medium for capturing and reflecting on one's experiences. It can also be used to explore themes of identity, memory, and perspective.

Integrating Art Therapy with Other Therapies

Art therapy can be effectively integrated with other therapeutic approaches, enhancing their efficacy:

Combined with Cognitive-Behavioral Therapy (CBT): Art therapy can help clients visualize cognitive distortions and practice new, healthier thought patterns.

Incorporated into Trauma-Focused Therapy: Art therapy provides a non-verbal way to process traumatic memories, making it a valuable tool in trauma-focused therapy.

Complementing Mindfulness Practices: Creating art can be a form of mindfulness, helping clients stay present and grounded.

Ethical Considerations

Ethical practice is crucial in art therapy. Therapists must ensure:

Confidentiality: Protecting clients' privacy and the confidentiality of their artwork.

Informed Consent: Ensuring clients understand the nature and purpose of art therapy.

Cultural Sensitivity: Being aware of and respectful towards the cultural backgrounds and practices of clients.

Professional Boundaries: Maintaining appropriate boundaries to foster a safe and therapeutic environment.

Conclusion

Understanding the theoretical foundations and therapeutic mechanisms of art therapy is essential for both practitioners and clients. By integrating psychological theories with creative expression, art therapy offers a powerful tool for healing and personal growth. The subsequent chapters will delve deeper into specific techniques, practical applications, and real-life success stories, providing you with a comprehensive guide to the transformative world of art therapy.

This chapter aims to provide readers with a thorough understanding of what art therapy is, its theoretical underpinnings, and how it functions as a therapeutic tool.

Chapter 3: The Healing Power of Art

Art therapy harnesses the profound connection between creativity and emotional healing. This chapter explores the various ways in which art can serve as a powerful tool for therapy, promoting mental and emotional well-being. We'll delve into the psychological and physiological mechanisms through which art facilitates healing, supported by case studies and real-life examples.

How Art Heals

The process of creating art can have multiple therapeutic benefits. It engages both the mind and body, offering a holistic approach to healing. Here are some key ways in which art contributes to emotional and psychological well-being:

Non-Verbal Expression: Art allows individuals to express feelings and thoughts that might be difficult to articulate verbally. This is particularly beneficial for those who have experienced trauma or who struggle with verbal communication.

Emotional Release: The act of creating art can be cathartic, providing an outlet for releasing pent-up emotions. The physical act of drawing, painting, or sculpting can help individuals process and let go of negative emotions.

Stress Reduction: Engaging in creative activities can induce a state of flow, where individuals become fully immersed in the task at hand. This state is associated with reduced stress and increased feelings of well-being.

Enhanced Self-Awareness: Creating art encourages introspection and self-reflection. Individuals can gain insights into their inner worlds, uncovering thoughts and feelings that might be hidden or suppressed.

Empowerment and Self-Esteem: Successfully creating a piece of art can boost self-esteem and a sense of accomplishment. It provides tangible evidence of one's abilities and creativity.

Mindfulness and Presence: The creative process encourages mindfulness, helping individuals stay present and focused. This can be particularly helpful for those dealing with anxiety and stress.

Psychological Mechanisms

Several psychological mechanisms underlie the therapeutic effects of art therapy:

Symbolic Representation: Art allows for the symbolic representation of thoughts and emotions. Through symbols and metaphors, individuals can explore complex feelings and experiences in a safe and manageable way.

Projection: The act of creating art can facilitate projection, where individuals unconsciously project their feelings and thoughts onto their artwork. This can provide valuable insights for both the client and therapist.

Containment: Art can serve as a container for difficult emotions, helping individuals manage overwhelming feelings. The boundaries of the artwork provide a safe space for exploring intense emotions.

Physiological Mechanisms

Creating art can also have positive effects on the brain and body:

Brain Activation: Art-making activates multiple areas of the brain, including those involved in sensory perception, movement, emotions, and cognition. This holistic brain engagement can enhance overall brain function and connectivity.

Stress Hormone Reduction: Engaging in creative activities has been shown to reduce levels of cortisol, a stress hormone. Lower cortisol levels are associated with reduced stress and improved immune function.

Neuroplasticity: The process of learning and creating new art can promote neuroplasticity, the brain's ability to reorganize itself by forming new neural connections. This can enhance cognitive flexibility and resilience.

Case Studies

To illustrate the healing power of art, let's explore some real-life examples:

Case Study 1: Emily's Recovery from Anxiety

Emily, a 28-year-old graphic designer, struggled with chronic anxiety. Through art therapy, she used drawing and painting to express her fears and worries. One of her most significant pieces was a series of drawings depicting her anxiety as a tangled web. As she worked through these drawings, Emily began to understand the roots of her anxiety and develop healthier coping strategies. The process of externalizing her internal struggles through art helped her gain control over her anxiety.

Case Study 2: John's Journey with PTSD

John, a 45-year-old military veteran, experienced severe PTSD after returning from deployment. Traditional talk therapy had limited success, so his therapist introduced art therapy as a complementary approach. John found solace in creating sculptures, using clay to mold and shape his traumatic memories. Over time, he created a series of sculptures that told his story of pain, resilience, and healing. This non-verbal expression allowed him to process his trauma in a new way, leading to significant improvements in his mental health.

Different Art Forms and Their Benefits

Different forms of art can have unique therapeutic benefits. Here are some examples:

Drawing and Painting: These forms allow for immediate and direct expression. The choice of colors, shapes, and lines can reveal a lot about a person's emotional state.

Sculpture and 3D Art: Working with three-dimensional materials can be particularly grounding and help individuals connect with their physical selves. It can also be a way to express and process more tactile or somatic experiences.

Collage and Mixed Media: Combining various materials and images can help individuals explore and integrate different aspects of their identity and experiences. Collage can be especially helpful for those who feel fragmented or are dealing with complex emotions.

Digital Art: Digital art offers endless possibilities for creativity and can be less intimidating for some individuals. It allows for easy experimentation and modification, which can be liberating for those who fear making mistakes.

Photography: Photography can be a powerful medium for capturing and reflecting on one's experiences. It can be used to explore themes of identity, memory, and perspective.

Integrating Art into Daily Life

Art therapy doesn't have to be confined to therapy sessions. Here are some ways individuals can incorporate art into their daily lives for ongoing emotional and psychological well-being:

Journaling with Art: Combining writing and drawing in a journal can be a daily practice for self-reflection and emotional expression.

Mindful Doodling: Simple doodling can be a form of mindfulness, helping individuals stay present and relaxed.

Creative Breaks: Taking short breaks during the day to engage in a creative activity, such as coloring or sketching, can reduce stress and enhance focus.

Art Projects: Engaging in larger art projects, such as creating a mural or a series of paintings, can provide a sense of purpose and accomplishment.

Conclusion

Art therapy leverages the healing power of creativity to promote mental and emotional well-being. By engaging in the creative process, individuals can explore and express their inner worlds, leading to greater self-awareness, emotional release, and psychological resilience. The next chapter will delve into specific techniques and methods used in art therapy, providing practical guidance for both therapists and individuals seeking to harness the therapeutic potential of art.

This chapter aims to provide a comprehensive overview of how art therapy works and its therapeutic benefits, supported by case studies and examples.

Chapter 4: Key Techniques and Methods

Art therapy employs a diverse range of techniques and methods to facilitate healing and self-expression. This chapter will explore various art forms and specific techniques used in art therapy, providing practical guidance on how to implement them. Whether you are an aspiring art therapist or an individual seeking to explore art therapy on your own, these techniques can offer valuable tools for emotional and psychological growth.

Drawing and Painting

Drawing and painting are fundamental techniques in art therapy, allowing for immediate and direct expression of thoughts and emotions.

Free Drawing:

Description: Encourages spontaneous drawing without a specific goal or outcome.

Purpose: To allow the unconscious mind to surface through unstructured expression.

How to Use: Provide clients with paper and a variety of drawing tools (pencils, markers, crayons) and invite them to draw whatever comes to mind.

Guided Imagery Drawing:

Description: Combines relaxation techniques with drawing to explore inner experiences.

Purpose: To access deeper layers of the psyche and uncover hidden emotions.

How to Use: Guide clients through a relaxation exercise, then ask them to draw an image that comes to mind during the process.

Emotion-Based Painting:

Description: Uses painting to express and explore specific emotions.

Purpose: To externalize and process complex emotions.

How to Use: Ask clients to choose a color that represents their current emotion and use it to create an abstract or representational painting.

Sculpture and 3D Art

Working with three-dimensional materials can be particularly grounding and provide a tactile way to express feelings and experiences.

Clay Modeling:

Description: Uses clay to create forms and shapes that represent inner experiences.

Purpose: To connect with physical sensations and express emotions through touch.

How to Use: Provide clients with clay and encourage them to mold it into shapes that represent their feelings or experiences.

Found Object Sculpture:

Description: Involves creating sculptures from everyday objects and materials.

Purpose: To explore themes of identity and transformation.

How to Use: Ask clients to collect objects that resonate with them and use them to build a sculpture that tells a story or represents an aspect of their life.

Assemblage Art:

Description: Combines various materials and objects into a cohesive artwork.

Purpose: To explore the integration of different aspects of the self.

How to Use: Provide a variety of materials (wood, metal, fabric) and encourage clients to create an assemblage that reflects their inner world.

Collage and Mixed Media

Collage and mixed media techniques allow for the exploration of identity and experiences through the combination of various materials and images.

Identity Collage:

Description: Uses cut-out images and text to create a collage that represents different aspects of the self.

Purpose: To explore and integrate various facets of identity.

How to Use: Provide magazines, scissors, and glue, and ask clients to create a collage that reflects who they are or how they see themselves.

Emotion Collage:

Description: Focuses on expressing emotions through the selection and arrangement of images and materials.

Purpose: To externalize and process emotions in a visual format.

How to Use: Ask clients to choose images and materials that represent their current emotional state and arrange them into a cohesive collage.

Mixed Media Self-Portrait:

Description: Combines different materials and techniques to create a self-portrait.

Purpose: To explore and express the complexity of the self.

How to Use: Provide various art supplies (paint, fabric, found objects) and encourage clients to create a self-portrait using mixed media.

Digital Art

Digital art offers endless possibilities for creativity and can be particularly appealing to those who are comfortable with technology.

Digital Collage:

Description: Uses digital tools to create collages from various images and graphics.

Purpose: To explore identity and experiences through digital media.

How to Use: Provide access to digital art software and guide clients in creating digital collages that reflect their inner world.

Digital Painting:

Description: Uses digital painting tools to create artwork.

Purpose: To express and explore emotions and experiences through digital media.

How to Use: Provide clients with a tablet or computer and digital painting software, and encourage them to create paintings that reflect their feelings or experiences.

Virtual Reality Art:

Description: Uses virtual reality (VR) tools to create immersive art experiences.

Purpose: To explore new dimensions of creativity and expression.

How to Use: Provide access to VR art tools and guide clients in creating virtual artworks that they can interact with in a three-dimensional space.

Photography

Photography can be a powerful medium for capturing and reflecting on one's experiences.

Photo Journaling:

Description: Combines photography with journaling to document and reflect on daily experiences.

Purpose: To promote mindfulness and self-reflection.

How to Use: Encourage clients to take daily photographs and write about their thoughts and feelings related to each image.

Themed Photo Projects:

Description: Focuses on specific themes or topics for photography projects.

Purpose: To explore and express specific aspects of life or identity.

How to Use: Ask clients to choose a theme (e.g., "Joy," "Change") and create a series of photographs that explore this theme.

Portrait Photography:

Description: Uses portrait photography to explore identity and self-perception.

Purpose: To examine and reflect on how individuals see themselves and how they are seen by others.

How to Use: Guide clients in taking or posing for portraits that reflect different aspects of their identity.

Integrating Techniques into Therapy

Combining various art therapy techniques can enhance the therapeutic process. Here are some ways to integrate these techniques effectively:

Sequential Art Making: Start with one technique (e.g., drawing) and then move to another (e.g., sculpture) to deepen the exploration of a theme or emotion.

Layered Approaches: Use multiple techniques in a single session, such as combining collage and painting, to provide a richer, more complex expression.

Thematic Sessions: Focus on a specific theme (e.g., "Transformation") and use different techniques to explore this theme from multiple angles.

Practical Tips for Implementing Techniques

When implementing art therapy techniques, consider the following tips to enhance the therapeutic experience:

Create a Safe Space: Ensure that the environment is welcoming and free from judgment, where clients feel safe to express themselves.

Encourage Exploration: Allow clients to experiment with different materials and techniques without worrying about the outcome.

Be Present: Offer your full attention and support during the art-making process, providing guidance as needed.

Reflect and Discuss: After the art-making, take time to discuss the process and the artwork, helping clients to gain insights and meaning from their creations.

Conclusion

Art therapy techniques and methods provide a versatile and powerful toolkit for facilitating healing and self-expression. By exploring various art forms and integrating them into therapy, both therapists and individuals can tap into the transformative potential of art. The next chapter will focus on applying these techniques to specific populations, tailoring approaches to meet the unique needs of children, adults, the elderly, and special populations.

This chapter aims to provide practical guidance on various art therapy techniques and methods, helping readers understand how to use these tools effectively in therapy or for personal growth.

Chapter 5: Tailoring Art Therapy for Specific Populations

Art therapy can be adapted to meet the unique needs of diverse populations. In this chapter, we will explore how to tailor art therapy techniques for children, adolescents, adults, the elderly, and special populations such as individuals with disabilities or those experiencing trauma. Each section will provide insights and practical tips for addressing the specific challenges and strengths of these groups.

Art Therapy with Children

Children are naturally expressive and often find it easier to communicate through art than through words. Art therapy can help them explore their emotions, develop social skills, and improve their self-esteem.

Techniques and Activities:

Storytelling and Drawing: Encourage children to draw pictures and then tell stories about their drawings. This helps them express their thoughts and feelings in a non-threatening way.

Puppet Making: Children can create puppets to act out scenarios or emotions, providing a safe distance from which to explore difficult feelings.

Emotion Faces: Use blank faces that children can draw on to express different emotions. This helps them identify and articulate their feelings.
Benefits:

Emotional Expression: Art therapy provides a safe outlet for children to express complex emotions.

Development of Motor Skills: Activities like drawing and cutting enhance fine motor skills.

Building Confidence: Successfully completing art projects can boost children's self-esteem.

Considerations:

Developmental Stage: Tailor activities to the child's developmental level.
Attention Span: Keep sessions short and engaging to match the child's attention span.
Parental Involvement: Involve parents in the process when appropriate, providing them with ways to support their child's artistic expression at home.

Art Therapy with Adolescents

Adolescents face unique challenges as they navigate the transition from childhood to adulthood. Art therapy can help them explore their identity, cope with stress, and build resilience.

Techniques and Activities:

Identity Collage: Adolescents can create collages that reflect their evolving sense of self.

Graffiti Art: Using graffiti-style art can appeal to teenagers and provide a rebellious yet safe form of self-expression.

Journaling with Art: Combining written journaling with drawings or doodles can help adolescents process their thoughts and emotions.
Benefits:

Self-Exploration: Art therapy provides a space for adolescents to explore and define their identity.

Emotional Regulation: Creating art can help adolescents manage stress and emotions.

Improved Communication: Art can serve as a bridge for adolescents to communicate with therapists and peers.

Considerations:

Autonomy: Respect adolescents' need for autonomy and provide choices in art activities.

Privacy: Ensure confidentiality to build trust.

Peer Influence: Be mindful of the influence of peers and address issues like peer pressure and social dynamics.

Art Therapy with Adults

Adults may seek art therapy to address a variety of issues, including mental health concerns, life transitions, and personal growth. Art therapy can help them explore their emotions, develop coping strategies, and enhance their well-being.

Techniques and Activities:

Mandala Creation: Drawing or coloring mandalas can promote relaxation and mindfulness.

Life Map: Clients can create a visual representation of their life journey, highlighting significant events and turning points.

Expressive Painting: Encourage adults to use painting as a way to express and process emotions.
Benefits:

Stress Relief: Engaging in creative activities can reduce stress and promote relaxation.

Insight and Reflection: Art therapy provides a means for adults to gain insights into their thoughts and behaviors.

Empowerment: Creating art can enhance self-efficacy and a sense of control.

Considerations:

Cultural Sensitivity: Be aware of and respect cultural differences in artistic expression and interpretation.

Trauma-Informed Care: Use trauma-informed approaches when working with individuals who have experienced trauma.

Goal Setting: Collaborate with clients to set realistic and meaningful goals for art therapy.

Art Therapy with the Elderly

Art therapy can support the mental and emotional well-being of elderly individuals, helping them cope with aging, memory loss, and physical limitations.

Techniques and Activities:

Reminiscence Art: Encourage elderly clients to create art that reflects their memories and life experiences.

Sensory Art Activities: Use tactile materials like clay or fabric to engage the senses.

Group Projects: Collaborative art projects can foster social connections and reduce feelings of isolation.

Benefits:

Cognitive Stimulation: Art-making can enhance cognitive function and memory.

Emotional Expression: Art provides a means for expressing feelings that might be difficult to articulate verbally.

Social Interaction: Group art activities can combat loneliness and promote social engagement.

Considerations:

Physical Limitations: Adapt activities to accommodate physical limitations and ensure accessibility.

Pace: Allow for a slower pace and be patient with the process.

Respect: Honor the life experiences and stories of elderly clients, using art to celebrate their legacy.

Art Therapy with Special Populations

Art therapy can be adapted to meet the needs of individuals with disabilities, those experiencing trauma, and other special populations.

Individuals with Disabilities:

Techniques and Activities: Use adaptive tools and materials to ensure accessibility. Focus on strengths and abilities rather than limitations.

Benefits: Art therapy can enhance communication, self-expression, and motor skills.

Considerations: Tailor activities to individual needs and provide a supportive, inclusive environment.

Trauma Survivors:

Techniques and Activities: Use trauma-informed approaches, such as creating safe spaces in art and focusing on grounding techniques.

Benefits: Art therapy can help process and integrate traumatic experiences, promoting healing and resilience.

Considerations: Be mindful of triggers and ensure a safe, supportive environment.

Groups and Communities:

Techniques and Activities: Facilitate community art projects or group sessions to foster connection and collective healing.

Benefits: Group art therapy can enhance social support, community cohesion, and collective resilience.

Considerations: Be sensitive to group dynamics and cultural contexts, ensuring inclusivity and respect for all participants.

Conclusion

Art therapy can be tailored to meet the unique needs of diverse populations, providing a versatile and powerful tool for healing and self-expression. By understanding the specific challenges and strengths of different groups, therapists can create meaningful and effective art therapy experiences. The next chapter will explore how to set up an art therapy practice, including practical considerations, ethical guidelines, and tips for creating a supportive and creative therapeutic environment.

This chapter aims to provide practical guidance on how to adapt art therapy techniques for various populations, addressing their specific needs and challenges.

Chapter 6: Setting Up an Art Therapy Practice

Establishing a successful art therapy practice requires careful planning, ethical consideration, and a supportive, creative environment. This chapter provides practical guidance on how to set up an art therapy practice, covering everything from choosing a location and acquiring materials to ethical guidelines and professional development.

Choosing a Location

Selecting the right location for your art therapy practice is crucial. Consider the following factors when choosing a space:

Accessibility:

Ensure that your location is easily accessible by public transport and has adequate parking facilities.

Make sure the space is accessible to individuals with disabilities.

Environment:

Choose a location that offers a quiet, private, and safe environment for clients. Consider the atmosphere of the space – it should be welcoming, comfortable, and conducive to creativity.

Space Requirements:

Ensure that you have enough space for individual and group sessions.
Include a separate area for storage of art materials and completed artworks.

Acquiring Materials and Setting Up the Space

Creating a well-equipped and inviting studio is essential for effective art therapy. Here are some tips on acquiring materials and setting up your space:

Essential Art Supplies:

Stock a variety of materials, including paints, brushes, pencils, markers, crayons, paper, canvas, clay, and collage materials.

Include both traditional and non-traditional art supplies to encourage creativity and exploration.

Furniture and Equipment:

Provide sturdy tables and comfortable chairs for clients to work on.
Ensure you have adequate storage solutions for art supplies and finished projects.

Consider investing in easels, drawing boards, and other specialized equipment as needed.

Creating a Therapeutic Environment:

Arrange the space to be welcoming and non-intimidating.
Include soft lighting, calming colors, and comfortable furnishings.
Display art pieces (with client consent) to create an inspiring and validating atmosphere.

Ethical Guidelines and Professional Standards

Adhering to ethical guidelines and professional standards is crucial in art therapy. Here are key considerations:

Confidentiality:

Ensure that client information and artwork are kept confidential.
Discuss confidentiality policies with clients at the outset and include them in consent forms.

Informed Consent:

Obtain informed consent from clients before starting therapy.
Ensure clients understand the nature of art therapy, its benefits, and any potential risks.

Boundaries and Safety:

Maintain professional boundaries to ensure a safe and respectful therapeutic relationship.

Be vigilant about creating a physically and emotionally safe environment for all clients.

Cultural Sensitivity:

Be aware of and respect cultural differences in art-making and expression.
Tailor your approach to meet the cultural and individual needs of each client.

Continuing Education:

Engage in ongoing professional development to stay updated on best practices and new developments in art therapy.
Participate in workshops, conferences, and peer supervision to enhance your skills and knowledge.

Marketing and Building Your Practice

Building a successful art therapy practice requires effective marketing and networking. Here are some strategies:

Networking:

Connect with other professionals in the mental health and healthcare fields. Join art therapy associations and local professional groups.

Online Presence:

Create a professional website that outlines your services, qualifications, and contact information.

Utilize social media to share insights, client testimonials (with consent), and examples of your work.

Community Engagement:

Offer workshops, presentations, or free introductory sessions to introduce art therapy to the community.

Collaborate with schools, community centers, and healthcare facilities to broaden your reach.

Client Referrals:

Establish referral relationships with other therapists, doctors, and community organizations.

Encourage satisfied clients to refer friends and family.

Managing Your Practice

Effective management is key to maintaining a thriving art therapy practice. Consider the following aspects:

Scheduling and Record Keeping:

Use scheduling software to manage appointments and reduce administrative workload.

Keep detailed records of client sessions, progress, and artwork (with consent).

Financial Management:

Set clear policies for fees, payment, and cancellations.

Consider using accounting software to manage your finances and track expenses.

Self-Care:

Prioritize self-care to avoid burnout and maintain your own well-being. Set boundaries between work and personal life, and seek supervision or therapy if needed.

Case Studies: Successful Art Therapy Practices

To provide inspiration and practical insights, here are some examples of successful art therapy practices:

Case Study 1: Creative Healing Studio

Overview: A small private practice that specializes in working with trauma survivors.

Key Strategies: Focuses on creating a safe and nurturing environment, uses a trauma-informed approach, and engages in community outreach to build a client base.

Case Study 2: Artful Aging Center

Overview: A practice dedicated to working with elderly clients, offering both individual and group sessions.

Key Strategies: Emphasizes reminiscence and sensory art activities, partners with local senior centers, and offers intergenerational art programs.

Case Study 3: Youth Art Therapy Collective

Overview: A collaborative practice focused on adolescents, providing a range of art therapy services in schools and community centers.

Key Strategies: Utilizes engaging and relevant art forms like graffiti art and digital media, provides workshops and group sessions, and collaborates with educational institutions.

Conclusion

Setting up an art therapy practice involves thoughtful planning, adherence to ethical guidelines, and ongoing professional development. By creating a supportive and creative environment, marketing your services effectively, and managing your practice efficiently, you can build a successful and impactful art therapy practice. The next chapter will explore advanced topics in art therapy, including integrating technology, working with specific therapeutic goals, and measuring the effectiveness of art therapy interventions.

This chapter aims to provide comprehensive guidance on establishing and managing an art therapy practice, covering practical, ethical, and professional aspects.

Do you need a professional degree to practice as an art therapist?

Yes, becoming a professional art therapist typically requires a specialized degree and certification. Here are the general steps and requirements:

Educational Requirements

Bachelor's Degree:

While specific undergraduate degrees are not strictly required, many prospective art therapists earn their bachelor's degrees in fields related to art, psychology, social work, or counseling.
Master's Degree in Art Therapy:

Most professional art therapists hold a master's degree in art therapy or a related field with a focus on art therapy. Accredited art therapy programs provide comprehensive education in psychology, counseling, and the therapeutic use of art.

These programs often include coursework in human development, psychological theories, art therapy techniques, and clinical practice.
Certification and Licensure

Certification:

In many countries, certification is offered by professional organizations. For example, in the United States, the Art Therapy Credentials Board (ATCB) offers certification as a Registered Art Therapist (ATR) and Board Certified Art Therapist (ATR-BC).
Certification generally requires completion of an accredited graduate program, supervised clinical experience, and passing a certification exam.

Licensure:

Licensure requirements vary by region but often include completing a master's degree, acquiring supervised clinical experience, and passing a state or national exam.

Some regions may have specific licenses for art therapists, while others might require licensure under broader mental health professional categories.

Clinical Experience

Supervised Clinical Hours:

As part of or following their graduate education, aspiring art therapists must complete a certain number of supervised clinical hours. This hands-on experience is critical for developing practical skills in applying art therapy techniques with clients.

Continuing Education

Ongoing Professional Development:

To maintain certification and licensure, art therapists are usually required to participate in continuing education. This ensures they stay updated on the latest research, techniques, and ethical standards in the field.

Professional Associations
Membership in Professional Organizations:
Joining professional associations, such as the American Art Therapy Association (AATA) or similar organizations in other countries, provides additional resources, networking opportunities, and professional support.

Legal and Ethical Considerations

Adhering to Ethical Standards:

Professional art therapists must adhere to ethical guidelines established by certifying bodies and professional organizations. This includes maintaining confidentiality, obtaining informed consent, and practicing within the scope of their training and expertise.

Conclusion

While a passion for art and helping others is essential, practicing as a professional art therapist requires formal education, certification, and adherence to ethical and legal standards. These requirements ensure that art therapists are well-equipped to provide effective and ethical therapeutic services to their clients.

Can you practice without a degree in Art Therapy?

Practicing as an art therapist without a formal degree in art therapy is generally not recommended and may be legally restricted in many regions. However, there are some alternative paths and roles you can consider if you are passionate about combining art and helping others but do not have an art therapy degree.

Alternative Paths

Art Facilitator or Instructor:

You can work as an art instructor or facilitator in community centers, schools, or recreational programs, using art to foster creativity and self-expression. While this is not therapy, it can have therapeutic benefits.

Therapeutic Art Activities:

You might lead therapeutic art activities in settings like nursing homes, hospitals, or community centers. In this role, you provide opportunities for participants to engage in creative activities without positioning yourself as a therapist.

Pursuing Related Fields:

If you have a degree in psychology, counseling, social work, or a related field, you could integrate art activities into your practice. However, you should be clear about your scope of practice and not claim to provide art therapy unless you have the appropriate credentials.

Volunteering and Non-Clinical Roles

Volunteering:

Volunteering at organizations that offer art therapy services can provide exposure and experience. While you won't be practicing as an art therapist, you can support the work of credentialed professionals.

Arts in Health Programs:

Many hospitals and healthcare facilities have arts in health programs that incorporate art-making into patient care. These programs often welcome volunteers and staff who can support patients in engaging with art, under the guidance of healthcare professionals.

Continuing Education and Workshops

Workshops and Short Courses:

Participating in workshops, short courses, and professional development programs related to art therapy can enhance your skills and understanding. Some programs offer certificates of completion, which can be useful for professional development.

Working Towards Certification

If you are committed to becoming an art therapist, you might consider the following steps to work towards the necessary qualifications:

Enroll in a Graduate Program:

Consider enrolling in a master's program in art therapy or a related field. Many programs offer flexible options for working adults, including part-time and online formats.

Gain Relevant Experience:

Work in related fields such as counseling, social work, or mental health support while pursuing your degree. This experience can be valuable when applying for art therapy programs and certification.

Legal and Ethical Considerations

Understanding Local Regulations:

Regulations regarding the practice of art therapy vary widely by region. It is important to understand the specific requirements and restrictions in your area to ensure that you are practicing legally and ethically.

Conclusion

While it is generally not possible to practice as a certified art therapist without a formal degree in art therapy, there are various ways to engage with therapeutic art activities and support others through creative expression. If you are passionate about this field, consider pursuing the necessary education and credentials to become a professional art therapist. This will not only enhance your ability to provide effective and ethical care but also open up more opportunities for professional growth and fulfillment.

Can I help general population to engage in art activities which work as therapy?

Yes, you can definitely help the general population engage in art activities that have therapeutic benefits, even if you are not a certified art therapist. While you cannot practice art therapy in a formal clinical sense without the necessary qualifications, you can still facilitate art activities that promote well-being and self-expression. Here are some ways to do this responsibly and effectively:

1. Facilitating Therapeutic Art Activities

Community Workshops and Classes:

Organize Workshops: Host art workshops in community centers, libraries, schools, or online. These can focus on different art techniques and encourage participants to express themselves creatively.

Themes and Projects: Create themed projects that explore emotions, stress relief, self-discovery, and personal growth. Activities like mandala drawing, vision boards, or expressive painting can be particularly therapeutic.

Support Groups:

Art for Self-Care: Start support groups where art-making is part of self-care practices. These groups can meet regularly to create art, share experiences, and support one another.

Focus on Process Over Product: Emphasize the process of creating art rather than the finished product. This approach helps participants focus on their experience and emotions during the creation process.

2. Creating a Safe and Supportive Environment

Establish Guidelines:

Respect and Confidentiality: Set ground rules that emphasize respect, confidentiality, and non-judgment. Participants should feel safe to express themselves without fear of criticism.

Inclusive Atmosphere: Ensure that your sessions are inclusive and welcoming to people of all backgrounds and abilities.
Materials and Accessibility:

Provide Various Materials: Offer a range of art supplies to cater to different preferences and abilities. This might include paints, markers, clay, collage materials, and digital art tools.

Adaptability: Be prepared to adapt activities for individuals with different needs, ensuring everyone can participate comfortably.

3. Incorporating Art into Daily Life

Personal Practice:

Encourage Daily Art: Promote the idea of keeping a daily art journal or sketchbook. This can help individuals process their thoughts and emotions regularly.

Art Breaks: Suggest taking short breaks during the day to engage in simple art activities like doodling or coloring to reduce stress.

Family and Group Activities:

Family Art Projects: Encourage families to engage in collaborative art projects, which can strengthen bonds and provide a shared, positive experience.

Community Art Initiatives: Organize community art projects, such as murals or collaborative installations, which can foster a sense of community and collective achievement.

4. Providing Resources and Guidance

Books and Online Resources:

Recommend Reading: Suggest books on art as a therapeutic practice, mindfulness, and creativity. Examples include "The Artist's Way" by Julia Cameron and "Drawing on the Right Side of the Brain" by Betty Edwards.

Online Tutorials: Share online resources, tutorials, and courses that guide individuals through various art techniques and projects.
Workshops and Seminars:

Invite Experts: Occasionally invite certified art therapists or mental health professionals to conduct workshops or seminars. This can provide participants with deeper insights and techniques.

5. Ethical Considerations

Clarify Your Role:

Transparency: Be clear about your qualifications and role. Make sure participants understand that while the activities may have therapeutic benefits, you are not providing clinical art therapy.

Referrals: Be prepared to refer individuals to licensed professionals if they need more intensive therapeutic support. Establish connections with local therapists and mental health professionals for this purpose.

Respect Boundaries:

Avoid Diagnosing: Do not attempt to diagnose or treat mental health conditions. Focus on the benefits of creativity and self-expression without delving into areas that require professional training.

Conclusion

By facilitating art activities that promote well-being and self-expression, you can make a positive impact on the general population. While it's important to stay within the boundaries of your expertise, you can still offer valuable opportunities for people to engage in creative processes that support their mental and emotional health. Always prioritize creating a safe, inclusive, and supportive environment for all participants.

Chapter 7: Advanced Topics in Art Therapy

Art therapy is a dynamic field that continues to evolve, incorporating new techniques, technologies, and theoretical frameworks. This chapter explores advanced topics in art therapy, delving into innovative approaches, specialized populations, and research-based practices.

Integrating Technology in Art Therapy

Technology has become increasingly integrated into the field of art therapy, offering new possibilities for creativity, accessibility, and connection.

Digital Art Platforms:

Explore the use of digital art software and apps as tools for art therapy. Virtual drawing and painting platforms can provide new avenues for self-expression, particularly for individuals who are comfortable with technology.

Virtual Reality (VR) Therapy:

Investigate the potential of virtual reality technology for immersive art therapy experiences. VR environments can simulate therapeutic settings, offer interactive art-making tools, and create virtual galleries for self-reflection.

Online Therapy Platforms:

Consider the benefits and challenges of providing art therapy through online platforms. Teletherapy allows for greater accessibility and convenience but may present limitations in terms of building rapport and interpreting nonverbal cues.

Specialized Populations and Settings

Art therapy can be tailored to meet the unique needs of specialized populations and settings, including clinical, educational, and community-based settings.

Medical Art Therapy:

Explore the role of art therapy in medical settings, such as hospitals, clinics, and rehabilitation centers. Art therapy can support patients coping with chronic illness, pain management, and adjustment to medical procedures.

Military and Veterans:

Examine the use of art therapy in working with military personnel, veterans, and their families. Art therapy can address issues related to trauma, PTSD, and the transition to civilian life, offering a creative outlet for expression and healing.

Forensic Art Therapy:

Discuss the application of art therapy in forensic settings, such as prisons, juvenile detention centers, and rehabilitation programs. Art therapy can help individuals in the criminal justice system explore issues related to identity, trauma, and rehabilitation.

Advanced Techniques and Approaches

Art therapists employ a variety of advanced techniques and approaches to deepen the therapeutic process and address complex issues.

Symbolism and Metaphor:

Explore the use of symbolism and metaphor in art therapy. Artwork can serve as a symbolic representation of inner experiences, allowing clients to explore unconscious thoughts and emotions.

Narrative and Storytelling:

Utilize narrative techniques to help clients create personal stories through art. Artwork can serve as visual narratives, allowing clients to externalize their experiences, reflect on their life journey, and explore new narratives.

Trauma-Informed Art Therapy:

Adopt trauma-informed approaches to art therapy, recognizing the impact of trauma on individuals' lives and relationships. Art therapy can provide a safe and supportive space for trauma survivors to process their experiences, build resilience, and reclaim their sense of agency.

Research and Evaluation in Art Therapy

Advancements in research and evaluation contribute to the evidence base for art therapy, informing best practices and enhancing the credibility of the field.

Outcome Studies:

Review outcome studies and research articles that examine the effectiveness of art therapy interventions across different populations and settings. Outcome measures may include improvements in mood, self-esteem, coping skills, and interpersonal relationships.

Qualitative Research Methods:

Explore qualitative research methods used in art therapy, such as thematic analysis, narrative inquiry, and phenomenological approaches. Qualitative research allows for in-depth exploration of clients' experiences and perspectives.

Art-Based Assessment Tools:

Investigate art-based assessment tools used in art therapy practice, such as the Draw-a-Person test, the House-Tree-Person test, and the Kinetic Family Drawing. These tools can provide insights into clients' thoughts, feelings, and relationships.

Professional Development and Supervision

Continuing education and supervision are essential for art therapists to stay informed, engaged, and effective in their practice.

Supervision and Consultation:

Seek supervision and consultation from experienced art therapists, psychologists, or counselors. Supervision provides a structured space for reflection, feedback, and professional growth.

Professional Conferences and Workshops:

Attend professional conferences, workshops, and training seminars to stay updated on current trends, research findings, and best practices in art therapy. These events offer opportunities for networking, learning, and collaboration with peers.

Publication and Presentation:

Share your expertise and insights through publication and presentation. Write articles for professional journals, contribute to books or edited volumes, and present at conferences or community events.

Conclusion

Advanced topics in art therapy encompass a wide range of innovative approaches, specialized populations, and research-based practices. By exploring these topics, art therapists can deepen their understanding of the field, refine their clinical skills, and contribute to the advancement of art therapy practice and research. Continued professional development, supervision, and engagement with emerging trends are essential for art therapists to provide effective and ethical care to their clients.

This chapter aims to provide insights into advanced topics in art therapy, offering a deeper understanding of innovative approaches, specialized populations, and research-based practices in the field.

Chapter 8: Cultivating Creativity and Self-Care

Creativity is at the heart of art therapy, serving as a powerful tool for self-expression, exploration, and healing. In this chapter, we explore strategies for cultivating creativity in both clients and therapists, as well as techniques for self-care to maintain well-being in the demanding field of art therapy.

Nurturing Creativity in Clients

As art therapists, fostering creativity in our clients is essential for facilitating meaningful therapeutic experiences.

Creating a Safe Space:

Establish an environment that encourages experimentation, risk-taking, and non-judgmental expression. Clients should feel free to explore their creativity without fear of criticism.

Embracing Process-Oriented Art:

Focus on the process of art-making rather than the end product. Encourage clients to enjoy the act of creating without worrying about producing a masterpiece.

Exploring Different Mediums:

Introduce clients to a variety of art materials and techniques, allowing them to discover which mediums resonate with them. Experimentation can spark new ideas and perspectives.

Encouraging Playfulness:

Foster a sense of playfulness and curiosity in clients' art-making processes. Play can unlock creativity and help clients tap into their imagination.

Creative Techniques and Exercises

Art therapists can employ a range of creative techniques and exercises to stimulate imagination, self-awareness, and personal growth.

Collage and Mixed Media:

Invite clients to create collages using found objects, photographs, and magazine clippings. Collage allows for spontaneous expression and the integration of diverse materials.

Expressive Movement:

Incorporate movement-based activities into art therapy sessions, such as dance, gesture drawing, or body mapping. Movement can evoke emotions and facilitate embodied expression.

Visual Journaling:

Encourage clients to keep visual journals as a means of self-reflection and exploration. Visual journaling combines writing with drawing, painting, or collage to capture thoughts, feelings, and experiences.

Storytelling and Narrative:

Invite clients to create visual narratives or tell stories through their artwork. Art can serve as a powerful storytelling medium, allowing clients to externalize their inner experiences.

Cultivating Creativity in Therapists

As art therapists, maintaining our own creativity is essential for effective practice and personal fulfillment.

Artistic Practice:

Make time for your own artistic practice outside of therapy sessions. Engaging in art-making nourishes creativity and provides a means of self-expression and reflection.

Continuing Education:

Stay curious and open to learning new techniques, theories, and approaches in art therapy. Attend workshops, conferences, and training programs to expand your knowledge and skills.

Peer Supervision and Collaboration:

Seek out opportunities for peer supervision and collaboration with other art therapists. Peer support can provide valuable feedback, inspiration, and validation.

Exploring Interdisciplinary Perspectives:

Draw inspiration from other disciplines, such as psychology, anthropology, or philosophy. Integrating diverse perspectives can enrich your understanding of art therapy and broaden your creative repertoire.

Self-Care Practices for Art Therapists

The demanding nature of the art therapy profession underscores the importance of self-care for therapists' well-being and effectiveness.

Mindfulness and Meditation:

Incorporate mindfulness and meditation practices into your daily routine to reduce stress, cultivate presence, and enhance self-awareness.

Physical Activity and Movement:

Prioritize regular exercise and physical activity to promote physical health and relieve tension. Movement-based practices like yoga or tai chi can also support emotional balance.

Setting Boundaries:

Establish clear boundaries between work and personal life to prevent burnout and maintain a healthy work-life balance. Schedule regular breaks and vacations to recharge and rejuvenate.

Seeking Support:

Reach out for support from colleagues, friends, and family members when needed. Cultivate a network of trusted individuals who can offer encouragement, empathy, and perspective.

Conclusion

Cultivating creativity in both clients and therapists is fundamental to the practice of art therapy. By fostering a supportive environment, embracing diverse techniques, and prioritizing self-care, art therapists can harness the transformative power of creativity to promote healing, growth, and well-being. As we nurture our own creativity and model self-care practices, we become more effective and authentic agents of change in the lives of our clients.

This chapter aims to explore strategies for nurturing creativity in both clients and therapists, as well as techniques for practicing self-care to maintain well-being in the demanding field of art therapy.

Chapter 9: Exercises and Activities

In this chapter, we'll delve into a variety of exercises and activities designed to facilitate self-expression, exploration, and healing through art therapy. These exercises can be tailored to meet the needs and interests of individual clients, groups, or communities.

1. Emotion Color Wheel

Objective: Explore emotions through color associations.

Instructions:

Provide clients with a blank color wheel template or ask them to draw their own. Assign each section of the color wheel to a different emotion (e.g., red for anger, blue for sadness, yellow for joy).

Invite clients to fill in each section of the color wheel with colors that represent how they feel when experiencing that emotion.

Discuss the connections between colors and emotions, exploring personal associations and cultural influences.

2. Five Senses Collage

Objective: Engage the senses to evoke memories and emotions.

Instructions:

Provide magazines, photographs, and other visual materials.
Ask clients to create a collage using images that represent each of the five senses (sight, sound, taste, touch, smell).

Encourage clients to reflect on the memories, emotions, and sensations evoked by each image as they assemble their collage.

Explore the significance of sensory experiences in shaping personal narratives and identity.

3. Mandala Drawing

Objective: Promote relaxation, mindfulness, and self-awareness.

Instructions:

Provide clients with circular templates or ask them to draw their own mandala outlines.

Invite clients to fill in the mandala with shapes, patterns, and colors that reflect their thoughts, feelings, and intentions.

Encourage clients to focus on the process of drawing and coloring, allowing thoughts and emotions to arise and dissipate without judgment.
Discuss the symbolism and significance of the mandala as a representation of wholeness and integration.

4. Body Mapping

Objective: Explore body awareness, self-image, and personal boundaries.

Instructions:

Provide large sheets of paper and drawing materials.
Ask clients to trace the outline of their bodies onto the paper, either lying down or standing against a wall.

Invite clients to fill in the body outline with images, symbols, or words that represent their physical sensations, emotions, and experiences.
Facilitate a discussion about body awareness, self-perception, and the relationship between physical and emotional well-being.

5. Guided Imagery Painting

Objective: Tap into the subconscious and promote insight and self-discovery.

Instructions:

Guide clients through a relaxation exercise to induce a state of deep relaxation and receptivity.

Invite clients to visualize a peaceful and safe place in their minds, such as a serene landscape or comforting space.

Encourage clients to paint or draw their visualization onto paper, allowing the imagery to flow spontaneously from their subconscious.

Facilitate a discussion about the symbolism, themes, and emotions present in the artwork, helping clients uncover insights and meanings.

6. Group Collage Project

Objective: Foster connection, collaboration, and shared meaning-making.

Instructions:

Provide a large canvas or poster board and an assortment of collage materials.

Divide participants into small groups and assign each group a theme or topic to explore through collage (e.g., community, resilience, growth).

Encourage groups to collaboratively create a collage that reflects their assigned theme, sharing materials, ideas, and creative decisions.

Facilitate a group discussion about the process of collaboration, the symbolism within the collages, and the shared meanings that emerge.

Conclusion

These exercises and activities are just a starting point for the rich and varied practice of art therapy. By engaging in creative expression, clients can tap into their inner resources, process emotions, and develop new insights and coping strategies. As art therapists, our role is to create a supportive and empowering environment that encourages clients to explore, create, and discover the transformative power of art.

This chapter provides a range of exercises and activities that can be adapted and tailored to meet the needs and interests of clients in art therapy sessions.

Chapter 10: Measuring Success and Progress

In this chapter, we will explore methods for assessing the effectiveness of art therapy interventions and tracking clients' progress toward their therapeutic goals. While the benefits of art therapy can be subjective and multifaceted, it is important to establish meaningful indicators of success to guide our practice and demonstrate the value of art therapy to clients, caregivers, and other stakeholders.

1. Establishing Therapeutic Goals

Before we can measure success, it's essential to establish clear and achievable therapeutic goals with our clients.

Collaborative Goal-Setting:

Involve clients in the goal-setting process, ensuring that goals are relevant, meaningful, and aligned with their needs and aspirations.

SMART Goals:

Use the SMART criteria (Specific, Measurable, Achievable, Relevant, Time-bound) to ensure that goals are well-defined and actionable.

2. Assessing Progress

Once goals are established, we can use various assessment methods to track clients' progress over time.

Observational Assessment:

Observe clients' behavior, verbalizations, and artwork during sessions to gauge changes in mood, self-expression, and engagement.

Client Self-Report:

Encourage clients to reflect on their experiences and progress through self-assessment tools such as mood scales, symptom inventories, or journaling.

Artwork Analysis:

Analyze clients' artwork to identify themes, symbols, and changes in style or content over time. Artwork can serve as a visual record of clients' progress and inner experiences.

Outcome Measures

In addition to qualitative assessments, we can use standardized outcome measures to quantify the impact of art therapy interventions.

Psychological Measures:

Administer standardized assessments of psychological functioning, such as the Beck Depression Inventory, State-Trait Anxiety Inventory, or Quality of Life Scale, to track changes in symptoms and well-being.

Art-Based Assessment Tools:

Utilize art-based assessment tools, such as the Formal Elements Art Therapy Scale (FEATS) or the Diagnostic Drawing Series (DDS), to evaluate specific aspects of clients' artwork and artistic development.

4. Client Feedback

Client feedback is a valuable source of information about the perceived benefits and effectiveness of art therapy.

Feedback Surveys:

Administer anonymous surveys or feedback forms to clients to gather their perspectives on the therapeutic process, goals, and outcomes.

Exit Interviews:

Conduct exit interviews or follow-up sessions to solicit clients' reflections on their overall experience in art therapy, including what they found helpful or challenging.

Collaborative Review and Reflection

Regularly review progress with clients to celebrate achievements, address challenges, and adjust goals and interventions as needed.

Progress Reviews:

Schedule regular check-in sessions to review clients' progress toward their goals, discuss any changes or developments, and revise treatment plans accordingly.

Celebrate Milestones:

Acknowledge and celebrate clients' achievements and milestones along their therapeutic journey, reinforcing their sense of agency, resilience, and growth.

6. Documentation and Communication

Accurate and thorough documentation is essential for tracking progress, communicating with other professionals, and maintaining ethical standards.

Clinical Notes:

Keep detailed clinical notes documenting each session, including observations, interventions, client responses, and progress toward goals.

Interdisciplinary Communication:

Collaborate with other professionals involved in clients' care, such as psychologists, psychiatrists, or social workers, to share information, coordinate treatment plans, and ensure continuity of care.

Conclusion

Measuring success and progress in art therapy requires a thoughtful and multidimensional approach that integrates qualitative and quantitative assessments, client feedback, and ongoing collaboration. By establishing clear therapeutic goals, tracking progress through observation and assessment, and engaging in reflective practice and communication, art therapists can demonstrate the effectiveness of their interventions and support clients' growth and well-being.

This chapter provides guidance on establishing therapeutic goals, assessing progress, and measuring success in art therapy practice, highlighting the importance of collaboration, reflection, and communication throughout the therapeutic process.

Chapter 11: Challenges and Considerations

While art therapy can be a deeply rewarding and transformative practice, it also presents unique challenges and considerations for both therapists and clients. In this chapter, we will explore some of the common challenges encountered in art therapy and strategies for navigating them with compassion, creativity, and resilience.

1. Resistance and Ambivalence

Clients may experience resistance or ambivalence toward art therapy for various reasons, including fear of self-disclosure, skepticism about the therapeutic process, or discomfort with creative expression.

Building Trust and Rapport:

Focus on establishing a trusting and supportive therapeutic relationship built on empathy, acceptance, and respect. Encourage open dialogue and validate clients' feelings and concerns.

Exploring Resistance:

Explore clients' resistance through gentle inquiry, acknowledging their feelings without judgment. Help clients identify underlying fears or barriers to engagement and collaboratively address them.

2. Emotional Intensity

Art therapy can evoke strong emotions and memories, which may be overwhelming or distressing for clients.

Creating Safety and Containment:

Establish a safe and contained therapeutic environment where clients feel supported and able to explore difficult emotions at their own pace. Use grounding techniques and coping strategies to manage emotional intensity.

Regulating Arousal States:

Teach clients self-regulation techniques, such as deep breathing, progressive muscle relaxation, or mindfulness practices, to manage heightened arousal states and promote emotional resilience.

Ethical Dilemmas

Art therapists may encounter ethical dilemmas related to confidentiality, boundaries, dual relationships, and cultural competence.

Ethical Guidelines:

Familiarize yourself with ethical guidelines and standards of practice for art therapy, such as those established by professional organizations like the American Art Therapy Association (AATA) or the British Association of Art Therapists (BAAT).

Consultation and Supervision:

Seek consultation and supervision from experienced art therapists or mental health professionals when faced with ethical challenges. Discuss potential courses of action and ethical considerations to ensure informed decision-making.

4. Cultural Sensitivity

Art therapists must be mindful of cultural differences, values, and beliefs that may influence clients' perceptions of art therapy and their preferences for artistic expression.

Cultural Humility:

Approach clients with humility, curiosity, and openness to learning about their cultural backgrounds and perspectives. Avoid making assumptions or imposing your own cultural values onto clients.

Adapting Interventions:

Adapt art therapy interventions to honor and respect clients' cultural traditions, symbols, and artistic preferences. Collaborate with clients to explore culturally relevant themes and materials.

Burnout and Self-Care

Art therapists may experience burnout due to the emotional demands of the work, vicarious trauma, and compassion fatigue.

Self-Care Practices:

Prioritize self-care practices that nurture your physical, emotional, and spiritual well-being. Engage in activities that replenish your energy, such as exercise, mindfulness, creative pursuits, and spending time in nature.

Boundaries and Work-Life Balance:

Establish clear boundaries between work and personal life to prevent burnout and maintain a healthy balance. Schedule regular breaks, vacations, and time for relaxation and leisure activities.

Conclusion

Navigating the challenges and considerations inherent in art therapy requires a nuanced understanding of clients' experiences, effective therapeutic skills, and a commitment to ongoing self-reflection and growth. By approaching challenges with compassion, creativity, and resilience, art therapists can foster healing, empowerment, and transformation in their clients and themselves.

This chapter provides insights into common challenges and considerations encountered in art therapy practice, along with strategies for addressing them with empathy, professionalism, and self-care.

Chapter 12: Future Directions in Art Therapy

The field of art therapy is continually evolving, influenced by advancements in research, technology, and societal changes. This chapter explores potential future directions for art therapy, highlighting emerging trends, innovative practices, and areas for further development.

1. Integrating Technology

The integration of technology in art therapy offers new tools and platforms for creative expression, accessibility, and therapeutic engagement.

Digital Art Tools:

Explore the use of digital drawing and painting software, virtual reality (VR), and augmented reality (AR) as mediums for art therapy. These tools can provide new avenues for creativity and engagement, particularly for tech-savvy clients.

Online Art Therapy:

Develop and refine teletherapy practices to provide art therapy services remotely. Online platforms can expand access to art therapy for clients in remote or underserved areas, offering flexibility and convenience.

Mobile Applications:

Utilize mobile apps designed for mental health and art-making to complement in-person sessions. These apps can offer guided activities, relaxation exercises, and creative prompts for clients to use between sessions.

2. Research and Evidence-Based Practice

Continued research is crucial for validating the effectiveness of art therapy and informing best practices.

Outcome Studies:

Conduct rigorous outcome studies to assess the impact of art therapy on various populations and conditions. Use quantitative and qualitative methods to capture a comprehensive picture of therapeutic benefits.

Neuroscience and Art Therapy:

Investigate the neural mechanisms underlying the therapeutic effects of art-making. Collaborate with neuroscientists to explore how art therapy influences brain function, emotional regulation, and cognitive processes.

Standardized Assessments:

Develop and validate standardized assessment tools tailored to art therapy. These tools can help measure progress, evaluate interventions, and provide data for research studies.

3. Expanding Access and Inclusion

Efforts to expand access to art therapy and promote inclusivity are essential for reaching diverse populations and addressing systemic barriers.

Community-Based Programs:

Establish community-based art therapy programs in schools, community centers, and non-profit organizations. These programs can serve marginalized populations, including low-income families, immigrants, and refugees.

Cultural Competence:

Enhance cultural competence in art therapy practice and training. Develop resources and curricula that address cultural diversity, equity, and inclusion, ensuring that therapists are equipped to work with clients from diverse backgrounds.

Advocacy and Policy:

Advocate for policies that support the recognition and funding of art therapy services. Engage with policymakers, professional organizations, and advocacy groups to promote the value and accessibility of art therapy.

Interdisciplinary Collaboration

Collaboration with other disciplines can enrich art therapy practice and expand its applications.

Integrative Health:

Collaborate with healthcare providers, including doctors, nurses, and occupational therapists, to integrate art therapy into holistic treatment plans. Art therapy can complement medical treatments and support overall well-being.

Education and Special Needs:

Work with educators and special education professionals to incorporate art therapy into school settings. Art therapy can support students with learning disabilities, behavioral challenges, and emotional needs.

Social Justice and Activism:

Partner with social workers, activists, and community organizers to address social justice issues through art therapy. Art can be a powerful tool for raising awareness, fostering resilience, and promoting social change.

5. Professional Development and Training

Ongoing professional development and training are essential for advancing the field of art therapy and ensuring high-quality practice.

Continuing Education:

Offer continuing education opportunities for art therapists to stay updated on new research, techniques, and best practices. Workshops, conferences, and online courses can facilitate lifelong learning.

Supervision and Mentorship:

Strengthen supervision and mentorship programs to support emerging art therapists. Experienced practitioners can provide guidance, feedback, and professional growth opportunities.

Certification and Accreditation:

Advocate for standardized certification and accreditation processes for art therapy programs. Ensure that training programs meet high standards of education, ethics, and clinical competence.

Conclusion

The future of art therapy is filled with possibilities for innovation, expansion, and impact. By embracing technological advancements, promoting research, expanding access, fostering interdisciplinary collaboration, and investing in professional development, the field of art therapy can continue to evolve and thrive. These efforts will enhance the ability of art therapists to support healing, growth, and transformation in diverse populations around the world.

This chapter aims to explore future directions in art therapy, highlighting emerging trends, innovative practices, and areas for further development to ensure the continued evolution and impact of the field.

Chapter 13: Resources and Further Reading

As you continue your journey in art therapy, having access to a variety of resources and further reading materials can deepen your understanding and enhance your practice. This chapter provides a curated list of books, articles, organizations, and online resources to support your ongoing learning and professional development.

Books

"Art Therapy Techniques and Applications" by Susan I. Buchalter

This comprehensive guide offers practical techniques and applications for using art therapy with different populations and settings.

"The Art Therapy Sourcebook" by Cathy Malchiodi

A foundational text that covers the basics of art therapy, including its history, principles, and various techniques.

"Handbook of Art Therapy" edited by Cathy Malchiodi

An edited volume featuring contributions from leading art therapists, covering a wide range of topics and approaches in art therapy.

"Art as Therapy" by Alain de Botton and John Armstrong

This book explores how art can be used as a tool for emotional and psychological well-being.

"Materials & Media in Art Therapy: Critical Understandings of Diverse Artistic Vocabularies" edited by Catherine Hyland Moon

A detailed exploration of the various materials and media used in art therapy and their therapeutic implications.

"Art Therapy and the Neuroscience of Relationships, Creativity, and Resiliency: Skills and Practices" by Noah Hass-Cohen and Joanna Clyde Findlay

This book delves into the neuroscience behind art therapy, offering insights into how creative processes can enhance emotional and relational health.

Articles and Journals

"The Arts in Psychotherapy"

A peer-reviewed journal dedicated to exploring the therapeutic use of the arts, including art therapy research, practice, and theory.

"Art Therapy: Journal of the American Art Therapy Association"

The official journal of the American Art Therapy Association, featuring research articles, case studies, and theoretical discussions.

"International Journal of Art Therapy"

A journal that publishes international research and practice in art therapy, offering diverse perspectives and approaches.

"Art Therapy: Trauma and Neuroscience" by Kathy Luethje (Journal Article)

An article that explores the connections between art therapy, trauma recovery, and neuroscience.

Professional Organizations

American Art Therapy Association (AATA)

The leading organization for art therapy professionals in the United States, offering resources, certification, and advocacy.
Website: www.arttherapy.org

British Association of Art Therapists (BAAT)

The professional organization for art therapists in the UK, providing training, support, and resources.
Website: www.baat.org

International Expressive Arts Therapy Association (IEATA)

A global organization that promotes the expressive arts as a therapeutic practice, including art, music, dance, and drama therapy.
Website: www.ieata.org

Online Resources

Psychology Today Art Therapy Directory

A directory of certified art therapists, including articles and resources related to art therapy.
Website: www.psychologytoday.com/us/therapists/art-therapy

Art Therapy Blog

A blog offering articles, tips, and resources related to art therapy practices and techniques.
Website: www.arttherapyblog.com

Creative Counseling 101

A resource for creative counseling techniques, including art therapy activities and exercises.
Website: www.creativecounseling101.com

YouTube Channels:

Channels like "Art Therapy with Creativity in Mind" and "The Virtual Art Therapy Studio" offer video tutorials, discussions, and demonstrations of art therapy techniques.

Workshops and Training Programs

Expressive Arts Therapy Training Programs

Many universities and institutes offer specialized training in expressive arts therapies. Look for programs accredited by relevant professional bodies. Online Courses and Webinars

Websites like Coursera, Udemy, and CreativeLive offer online courses in art therapy and related fields. Check for courses that provide continuing education credits (CEUs).

Professional Conferences

Attend conferences such as the AATA Annual Conference or the IEATA Conference to network, learn from experts, and stay updated on the latest research and practices in art therapy.

Conclusion

These resources and further reading materials are designed to support your ongoing development as an art therapist. Whether you are seeking to deepen your knowledge, explore new techniques, or stay current with research and best practices, these books, articles, organizations, and online platforms offer valuable tools for growth and inspiration in your art therapy journey.

This chapter provides a comprehensive list of resources and further reading to support continuous learning and professional development in the field of art therapy.

As we reach the end of "The Art of Healing: Exploring Art Therapy for Personal Growth and Emotional Well-Being," I hope you feel inspired and empowered by the transformative power of art therapy. Throughout this journey, we've explored the profound ways in which creative expression can facilitate healing, enhance self-awareness, and foster emotional well-being.

Art therapy is more than a set of techniques; it's a dynamic and evolving practice that meets each individual where they are. Whether you are a practitioner, a student, or someone exploring art therapy for personal growth, remember that the essence of this work lies in its ability to connect us to our most authentic selves.

Here are a few key takeaways as you move forward:

Embrace the Process: The journey of art therapy is as important as the outcomes. Allow yourself to explore and create without judgment. The act of making art is itself a healing and insightful process.

Stay Curious: Continue to learn and explore new methods, materials, and approaches. The field of art therapy is rich with possibilities, and there is always more to discover.

Practice Self-Compassion: Be gentle with yourself as you navigate your emotions and experiences through art. Healing is a gradual process, and each step forward, no matter how small, is significant.

Connect with Others: Share your journey with others who can support and inspire you. Whether through professional networks, art therapy groups, or personal relationships, connections can provide invaluable insights and encouragement.

Reflect and Grow: Take time to reflect on your experiences and the artwork you create. Journaling, discussing your work with a therapist, or simply meditating on your creations can deepen your understanding and enhance your growth.

Advocate for Art Therapy: Spread awareness of the benefits of art therapy in your community. Advocate for its inclusion in schools, healthcare settings, and mental health services to make this valuable resource accessible to more people.

As you close this book, I encourage you to carry forward the principles and practices of art therapy in your daily life. Let creativity be a source of healing, joy, and discovery. Trust in the process, and know that through art, you have a powerful tool to navigate life's challenges and celebrate its beauty.

Thank you for joining me on this journey. May your path be filled with color, creativity, and healing.

With gratitude and hope,

Shazia Naqib

www.ingramcontent.com/pod-product-compliance
Lightning Source LLC
Chambersburg PA
CBHW082218220526
45470CB00010B/3217